CONTENTS

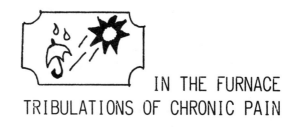

IN THE FURNACE
TRIBULATIONS OF CHRONIC PAIN

Please Hold our Umbrellas
When Doubts Rain Down
Upon our Spirits

*Contemplations for Those with Chronic
Pain or Experiencing Chronic Illness*

PRISCILLA OLSON

Published by Morris Publishing
3212 East Highway 30, Kearney,
Nebraska 68847

ISBN: 1-57502-068-8

Library of Congress Catalog Card Number: 95-92623

Printed in the USA by

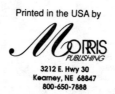

3212 E. Hwy 30
Kearney, NE 68847
800-650-7888

This book is dedicated to my
husband, Gordon, for his
love and unselfish support,
care giving, and understanding.

It is also dedicated to my Support Group members who boost
my spirits, love me, and will
me to be whole. It is dedicated, as well, to all Persons
with visible, or invisible,
chronic pain or chronic illness
who struggle daily to stand
firm in the midst of the fire.

FOREWORD

Life holds many blessings left unnoticed until something calls our attention to them.

I've never suffered chronic pain. And I took that for granted until I met individuals who were in its grip. I then learned to say thank you for my little aches and passing hurts, and to count my blessings differently than before.

I've noticed that persistent pain, with its brutal and unrelenting fetters, produces different results in the lives of its captives. Just as the same sun hardens the clay and melts the ice, so chronic pain has a way of revealing true character. Some become embittered and angry; their souls parched with their lot. Others develop into deep, cool springs of proven maturity and provide spiritual refreshment to those near them. The former raise a fist of defiance; the latter fold their hands in prayer.

That's what this book is about. In language of the soul, the author journals what pain has taught. She narrates its lessons with a sprinkling of humor, so characteristic of her personality.

I have also observed her husband, Gordon, endure his own pain; incessant in its own way. They walk this road together into an uncertain future, yet with deep trust in the One who has set the course and walks with them.

"Fear not; for I have redeemed thee, I have called thee by thy name; thou art mine. When thou passest through the waters, I will be with thee; and through the rivers, they shall not overflow thee; when thou walkest through the fire, thou shalt not be burned, neither shall the flame kindle upon thee. For I am the LORD thy God, the Holy One of Israel, thy Savior...." (Isaiah 43:1b-3a)

Pastor Galen Call
Grace Church Roseville

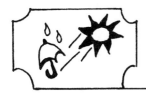

INTRODUCTION

"I believe in the sun even when it
is not shining; I believe in love
even when I feel it not: I believe
in God, even when He is silent."
(Found on a concentration camp wall.)

Putting words down frees our feelings from out
of the locked prison cells of our souls. We gain
objectivity and clarity through daily   journaling.
We find faith, courage, and regeneration of mind
and spirit.   This is a book about the furnace of
infirmity when the illness is raging, the pain is
rampant, and the future is seemingly lost in the
flames and smoke. The heat generated by the licking
flames underscores the limited power those of us
with chronic pain or chronic illness have over our
physical lives.   It is only when we locate the escape latch, replace   terror, dread, and fear with
true peace, stillness, and contentment of God's
sovereignty and Lordship that we are protected from
being consumed by the infernal trials and testings
of the oven.

We grieve for we have an unendurable sense of loss,
overwhelming sadness and loneliness, and feelings
of rejection, abandonment, disillusionment, and anxiety. We struggle. We   get stuck. We struggle
again. We   surrender and accept what we can not
change, but we do not give up. Many of us choose
to love God even when knowing that choice involves
chronic pain or illness which may mean forever - a
trial by fire.

No illness is truly acceptable to society, the least of all, an invisible illness. Diseases and pain that are chronic are not always manifest externally. Those of us suffering horrific, disabling pain that exists in and of itself, regardless of medication, pain management techniques, or rest, are not likely to receive support, compassion, nor understanding, because the symptoms are not obvious to the observer. They are a myriad of subjective, invisible, typically transient, unmeasurable symptoms that exacerbate and remit. Many of us experience them as chronic pain, chronic fatigue, transient visual disturbances, subtle transient memory loss, cognitive difficulties, muscular weakness, imbalance or difficulty with coordination, sleep disorders, speech impairment, transient bladder and bowel dysfunction, personality changes, and emotional liability. Many of us have nerve, neck, or back injuries. Others of us experience the challenges of MS, ALS, Lupus, Fibromyalgia, Sjogens, Raynaud's, Lymes, Vulvodynia, Post Polio Syndrome, HIV, Migraines, Endometreosis, Arthritis, degenerative conditions, and any of a number of other conditions, or "orphan" diseases.

Many of our symptoms defy medical measurement because they are subjective - and we look so well. Thus, when we see doctors, who are trained in scientific data, they most often are unable to observe any perceptible problem. We no longer are surprised to find these doctors bent on disproving the possibility of our symptoms without definitive laboratory tests. Minimal, or borderline, readings are discarded as being of insignificance. Our pain is a fact! Other's assessments are opinions. A lab test, or an x-ray, can not tell the intensity of ones pain. This relegates many of us to the vulnerability of being described as being under great stress, depressed, neurotic or psychosomatic. However, if the truth were to be known, any psychological problems that may exist may well have been caused by the anxiety of the failure of the medical profession to correct the painful, frustrating illness, to curb the pain, and to genuinely care.

It is a known fact that objective measurement can not measure the degree of subjective pain or fatigue, but "Damage to the body causes diminution of the self, which is further magnified by debasement of others." (Robert F. Murphy) Many times there are those among our number who are victimized by subtle, and often times not so subtle but very direct skepticism, ridicule, and criticism by doctors. The impossible trick we must perform in this medical merry-go-round is two-fold. First, we must have symptoms that are always constant, specific, uncomplicated, visible, and severe enough to be readily observable at all times. Second, we must have a doctor who is interested enough to take a full history with compensation for our transient memory loss and cognitive difficulties. He needs to be willing to review our own observations as noted in our medical diaries. In addition, he should assign us to read available research that is specific to our symptoms and provide him with a copy with pertinent areas highlighted, to save him time. He must be willing to continue to examine all the data beyond the 5-10 minutes allotted to each of us per office visit. Here in lies part of the problem. Our physician needs to be persistent, caring, and committed to follow each of us up; to outline ways of coping and combating the disease or condition that may be quite intangible; and to provide information, education, and options. By involving us in a search for knowledge, the Unknown becomes less frightening, stress is reduced, and we are offered hope to feel well. Our energy becomes directed into learning how to cope - letting the present moment be truly nourishing. Above all, our doctor needs to care, offer hope, and inspire confidence and optimism.

Pain is known by young and old alike. Pain is understood in any dialect or language. For most of us, pain is something that invades most of each hour of the day; yet, not understood. "But, you look just fine!" Thus, involvement in a Support Group is very important. We need a safe environment to share our pain, fear, and anger, as well as to share the more socially unacceptable symptomologies that engender shame, or embarrasment, or unbelief, if shared in public. A support group finds answers for us when pain is like a closed information booth. When we are a member of a group, we are not alone with our pain. Our common experiences are like a family quilt with each square telling our story. Being with others who know what pain is helps us to build strength, courage, and a will to endure, and cope.

When our lives flirt with the edge, and the daily ordeal of living with pain wears us down, a couple of hours in a Support Group helps restore a sense of control, and promotes positive change in behavior. A Support Group is not a replacement for acceptance in larger society. It is a lifeline of empathetic, nuturing, and caring people. Care and love increase tolerance to pain, and enhance recovery. A Support Group is not a frill. Participation is an essential part of our healing process. Our wellness depends on outside connections with support, listening, acceptance and caring by others in similar circumstances. We learn that when we have done our best and have actively participated in our care, to wait the results in peace.

Some of us remember the old pot-bellied, cast iron furnaces from our youth. They held a red hot fire for a very long time if banked well. We experience so much anger in pain. We bank our furnaces well. Our anger can not be changed until it is faced. Those of us with chronic pain or chronic illness can mobilize and use the energy signaled by our anger. We can turn anger's challenges into accomplishments. We must search for the meaning of our pain with the hope of making some peace with it; letting the burned out ashes fall through the grate and the tray to be emptied in the refuse pile. We may find that a rock bottom surrender is the best solution. We can be assured that God will keep His hand on "the damper system" while He waits for us to trust His plans for our ultimate good.

Many an inferno begins by the igniting of a match, but some begin by creosote buildup, or by a chimney fire. Yet fire can smolder in a log, or in a bed of coal, for a long time before erupting. Every one of "our fires" has had a beginning. For me, a Mixed Connective Tissue Disease touched off more than three decades of flickering and smoldering. However I believe this most fierce, raging fire errupted in late fall, 1989, resulting from a physical assault by a student in the high school at which I taught. He ran from in back of me and leaped with his full weight on my head and shoulders. Being seated, my spine, no doubt, was forced into my chair. This fire flared, and then extinguished, ever more frequently from early 1990 to 1992. Flames nearly consumed 1993 and 1994. This Pudendal Nerve Neuropathy and Urinary Disorder continue to rage into 1995. No one has been able to intercede. The burning quite literally, can not be quenched. A stint in the furnace changes the entire course of our lives. In spite of all the "modern extinguishers," pain rages on and hope seems to be enveloped in the rising smoke.

The burning, and our relentless pain or illness, may remind some of us of the Biblical account in Daniel where King Nebuchadnezzar heated a furnace 7 times hotter than usual. This was to consume three bound men - Shadrach, Meshach, and Abednego. Scripture says, "But lo, FOUR men were found walking in the midst of the fire, and the fourth appeared as like that of the Son of God." (Daniel 3:10-30)

When we have come to the end of ourselves, those of us with chronic pain or illness are given strength to believe that the Great Physician walks with men still in their furnace of tribulation. If we are persistent in our faith, we too will come forth from the midst of "our fire."

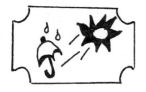

PAIN'S SIMILES

"If it is well with your belly, your back, and your feet, regal wealth can add nothing greater."

— Horace

PAIN IS LIKE SPAGHETTI

Pain is like stringy spaghetti;
Long, drawn out, and slippery,
Hidden in blood-red sauce,
Only made edible accompanied by meat balls.

Disguised in hot dish after hot dish,
With this condiment, or a little of that;
Combined pasta shapes in tossed salad,
Reserved daily from refrigerated containers.

Wormed
  Noodled
    Elbowed
      Shelled

PASTA IS PASTA BY ANY NAME!
Ever present on the Grocer's shelf
Twenty-four hours
Day, Night, Dawn.

PAIN IS LIKE A STALK OF CORN

Pain is like a stalk of corn;
Fertilized with Scotts
Enriched by Miracle Grow
-Sturdy and Strong-

Ears are shucked, eaten, or frozen;
Kernels canned whole, or creamed
-Useful-

Gray smut oozes from the stalk;
Cut worms hide in cobs
-Invaded-

Fires are lit, stoked, and fed;
A Gardener's effort consumed
-Destroyed-

Plight disregarded, slighted, over looked;
Extinguishers in hand not acknowledged
-Oblivious-

Smut
Worms
Fire
Indifference
Pain

PAIN IS LIKE A JUMP ROPE

Pain is like a jump rope;
  Round and round
    Keep in Step.
Whirling and twirling
    Skip in, skip out.
Swinging high, swooping low
    Hop to the beat.

Controlled by the Rotaters;
  Caught and dependent,
Condemned to their gyration;
  Doomed and degraded.

Give in to their pivot;
  Resist and agonize.
  Round and round
    Keep in step.
Whirling and twirling
    Skip in, skip out.

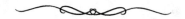

PAIN IS LIKE A BAG OF RICE

Pain is like a bag of rice;
   each grain a moment,
      but together,
an hour, a day, a month, or a year;
   Camouflaged in casseroles
with cream of chicken soup
     and mushrooms.

     CAUGHT
in the medical soup of indecision
   with pain mushrooming.

     RELIEF
disguised only for a time.

   THEN THROWN OUT
  with the left overs.

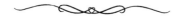

PAIN IS LIKE BUBBLE GUM

Pain is like bubble gum;
Many sticks to knead
with challenging massage;
Then, thrusting into air balls
-Vast, colossal, prodigious-
Bubbles with vulnerability
Stamina exhausted
Validity questioned
Soundness disputed
Perseverance tried.

The bubble blankets and obscures;
Encompassing and concealing
the effort of the fighter.
"Keep up the good work" bystanders shout
-Goading, Proding, Picking-
Renewed strains detonate the bubble;

Potentiality splattered
Confidence dampened
Success unrealized
Pain unabated.

PAIN IS LIKE A TYPEWRITER

Pain is like a typewriter
with a story to reveal,
But
Letters
are not positioned to foretell,

Words
are not descriptive enough,

Sentences
are not sufficiently expressive,

Paragraphs
are not adequately reflective,

Histories
are not convincingly credible;

Extinguished
Invalidated
Squelched
Squashed
Crushed
if not letter perfect
to the established code.

PAIN IS LIKE A PAIR OF PLIERS

Pain is like a pair of pliers
   locked in place
      gripping
         pinching
            tightening
            crushing
               dominating
                  mastering!

PAIN IS LIKE WINDEX

Unremitting pain is like Windex;
   Wiping away
Many little things, careers, and dreams.
   Sprayed on
Wiped clean
   No streaks
Obliterating existence.

PAIN IS LIKE A RUBBER BAND

Pain is like a rubber band...it
    stretches and reaches
        into every retreat;
    binds tightly and infringes
        on everything,
    destroys self-esteem,
    necessitates and compels one
        to beg for relief,
    shoots and snaps sharply,
        forces one to bear the sting,
    accumulates piles of
        medical bills,
    bursts, shatters, becomes
        pulverized, and
    leaves chances of a cure,
        a ruptured fissure.

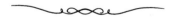

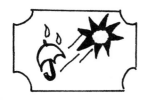

WHAT COLOR IS PAIN?

"Grace comes into the soul,

As the morning sun into the world:

First a Dawning:

Then a light:

And at last the sun in his full and

Excellent Brightness."

- Thomas Adams

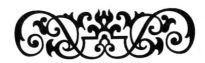

PAIN IS A BRUSH

Pain is a brush
  filled with brightest hues;
Streaking across the canvas,
  illustrating various views.

Pain is a brush
  inundated with brown and black;
Clouding figures on the canvas,
  obscuring what images lack.

Pain is a brush
  confused by color selection;
Streaking stripes and clashing shapes,
  applying pigment on an unwanted collection.

Pain is a brush
  dipped in varigated shade;
Reflecting willingness to compromise,
  repainting the discolorations made.

PAIN DICTATES THE COLOR

Pain is minus the color
and
   promise
      of the rainbow.

Pain thrusts coal black
   darts
      of misery
         and woe.

Pain showers a grey
   zigzagging
      electrical
         flow.

Pain is a blanket of white
   cold and smothering,
      choking the spirit's
         stow.

Pain is dark and devoid of light
   daring
      the sun to break through
         and grow.

WHAT COLOR IS PAIN?

What color is pain, if -
Yellow
　　is a window of promise?
White
　　is assurance of a miracle?
Green
　　is energy for tomorrow?
Red
　　is strength for today?
Pink
　　is hope in the future?
Orange
　　is a pledge for a pain-free day?
Brown
　　is a warranty of recuperation?
Purple
　　is an oath of wonder and marvel?
Blue
　　is a declaration of divine healing?
Black
　　is the absence of all that is good?

I TRY NOT TO SEE BLACK

I try not to see black when the storm rages;
Nor the purple and green billowing clouds,
Nor the grey funnels dropping to the ground,
Where hopes and dreams lie smashed and uprooted.
I strive to keep the pain under control.

I try not to hide in the dark overcast;
Nor in sunless, black places in life,
Nor in the ominous, threatening future,
Where only shadowy, obscure colors occur.
I strive to keep the pain under control.

I try not to believe in dingy, colorless diagnoses;
Nor in gloomy, sinister predictions,
Nor in somber, disheartening scenarios,
Where absence of light sullens the spirit.
I strive to keep the pain under control.

-I Try Not to See Black-

A GARMENT OF YELLOW

Lord, I know your hand holds the needle;
Steel poised above the fabric of my life.
   I wonder, may I kindly ask,
Will you please choose a lot of yellow?

Lord, I know you walked upon the water;
Lessons of power woven into my tapestry.
   Do you mind if I inquire,
Can you please use a lot of yellow?

Lord, I know you made water into wine;
Miracles of promise stitched into my material.
   Would you be offended if I ask,
Do you plan to utilize "a bunch" of yellow?

Lord, I know you stilled the storms at sea;
Confidence sewn into my article of cloth.
   Could I kindly request,
Would you put in some extra yellow?

Lord, you healed the sick and made the blind to see;
Divine marvels are hemmed in around my twill.
   If it's okay, may I ask,
Would you please go real heavy on the yellow?

Lord, I know you said to ask and I would receive;
Faith to be healed embroidered in my textile.
I wonder, may I respectfully ask,
Could you, by any chance, have forgotten the yellow?

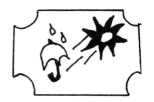

"I am not now that which
I have been."
- George Gordon Byron

"All things change, creeds and
philosophies and outward
systems, but God remains."
- Mary Augusta Ward

TATTERED REMAINS

Pain is like a shirt
   on washday;
   Securely fastened on the line;
Puffed, billowed, swollen
   by the summer's breeze.

Suddenly heavy gusts of wind
   involuntarily sweep
   on the quieted scene;
Ripping, tearing, shredding
   renting at the seams.

Colorful, tattered scraps
   fight so gallantly;
   giving in to the forceful gale,
Relenting, Submitting, acquiescing,
   only fragments of yesterday.

▴▴▴▴▴▴▴▴▴▴▴▴

PAIN IS MATHEMATICAL

The minuend of meaningful life-
The subtrahend of disease and pain
    withdraws
    withholds
    deducts
    subtracts
    minuses
The results being humungous losses,
    each needing grieving and resolution.

The dividend of quality life-
The divisor of pain and disease
    disunites
    partitions
    isolates
    detaches
    severs
Leaving a quotient-
    a small division of what was,
    and a small remainder.

GHOSTLY SILENCE MY COMPANY

Pain is so lonely, Lord,
Removed from the mainstream;
No longer included
Decisions reached without me.

Pain is so lonely, Lord,
Reminiscent of putting
  my hand in a bucket of water;
    Its trail
      My significance.

Pain is so lonely, Lord,
Plans and goals hewn down;
Replaced by modest saplings
Real living placed on hold.

Pain is so lonely, Lord,
Minutes tick into hours;
  Hours into days
    Ghostly silence my company.

Pain is so lonely, Lord,
The phone stops ringing;
  The doorbell fails to sound.
    The bucket of water
      Unchanged.

HELD BONDAGE TO PAIN'S ANGUISH

The torturous thief steals through the night;
A hideous predator devouring trust and certainty;
Dumping hope into a fathomless pit;
Abandoning control and increasing vulnerability.

A long journey of torment and agony;
  Minutes ticking as hours;
Held bondage to anguish that knows
  No length, nor breadth, nor height,
Forcing isolation accentuated with sadness;
  Yawning in a chasm of informational drought.

An island of heartache, woe, and grief;
Doctors blind to the extent of suffering;
Suspecting, disbelieving, questioning;
Vexing the soul, disallowing personal beliefs.

PAIN OUTBREAKING, SAVAGELY
RUNNING WILD

Pain is dry timber on a hot
   windswept day;
Igniting with the suggestion of a spark.
Flames raging, stinging, burning,
    licking;
All attempts to quench are rebuffed.

Coals smolder
    all the night long;
Fanning life in the long
    smog filled dawn;
Outbreaking, savagely running wild.

Then tamed
    for the moment;
Stirring restlessly,
    piercing the calm;
Acre after acre sorched and charred.

   Yet,
      Cunningly,
         Pain Sears
            In the underground bog.

PAIN CONTROLS THE STRINGS

The Puppeteer tries, but
PAIN

C			D
O		S	I
N	T	T	C
T	H	R	T
R	E	I	A
O		N	T
L		G	I
S		S	N
			G

"Its Every Move"

Deleting
    self-esteem at will;

Resistance
    crumpling its limbs;

Controlling
    each and every scene.

SOMETIMES I CRY

I see you stately, perennial birch tree
Standing so tall and staunch in the woods;
Your white paper bark and
   Conspicuous black triangles
      Mesmerize me.

Collectively you seduce and enchant me
I see parallels in our lives;
   Both growing, reaching,
Originating from an original
      Stem;
Growing hard and strong,
But simple and shy,
     And Dying; ·
Like your gold painted leaves in the Fall;
     Yet,
Having scattered and blown
  Minute winged nutlets
     To the next generation, just
As I have planted and instilled
    Knowledge, Understanding,
      And love.

    SEEDS planted on hearts of children
    BLOSSOMS nourished with joy
      FRUITS harvested with the "gift of reading"

    -My Legacy-

You have many uses
>Resins for tanning
>Oil and tar used medicinally
>Veneer finishes
>Furniture
>Toothpicks
>Construction
>Tepees, canoes, and sleds
>>Used by our common ancestors.

I have many roles
>Friend
>Wife
>Lover
>Teacher
>Mother
>Grandmother
>Crafter
>>Needed in many ways.

We are alike; We can't deny it.
>Short-lived
>Vulnerable
>Hewn down
>Desapped
>Peeled like an onion;
>>-Sometimes we cry-

THE STRUGGLE

"Suffering will either be your master or your servant, depending on how you handle the crisis of life. A crisis doesn't make a person. It reveals what a person is made of."

— Warren Wiersbe

PAIN HAS GREATER DEPTHS THAN A
FATHOMLESS SEA

God of early mornings
God of late nights
God of the mountain peaks
God of the seas
  - Be my God -

My pain has -
    horizons further away than early mornings
    deeper darkness than the nights of the earth
    higher peaks than arduous mountains
    greater depths than fathomless seas

God of the early mornings free my
    mind of pain so I can pray.
God of the late nights release the
    incessant burning so I can pray.
God of the mountain peaks stabilize
    the steep pathway of pain so I can pray.
God of the seas calm the stormy waves
    of pain so I can pray.

  - Be my God -

FATHER, I STRUGGLE

Father, I struggle each day;
Your path seems too arduous.
I feel so alone picking my way.
Rocks, mudslides, and washouts restrict.
Pain wracks my every move.

Father, I strive with valiant effort;
Your way seems too precarious and difficult.
I feel so exhausted trying so hard.
Storms, trials, and omens suppress.
Pain destroys my sense of hope.

Father, I fight to stay on the trail;
Your grade seems excessively steep.
I feel so discouraged and degraded.
Doctors, pain clinics, specialists invalidate.
Pain annihilates my every breath.

Father, I zealously exert 150 per cent;
Your course seems too overwhelming.
I feel so badgered and beaten down.
Questions, tests, annul my person.
Pain terrorizes and devastates my being.

Father, I need to walk in your foot steps;
Your imprints to lead my way.
I feel so vulnerable to the crows.
Silence, deafness, and secretiveness cause despair.
Pain rages, and ravages my existence.

I STRUGGLE WITH YOUR JUSTICE, GOD

My prayers are laced with loneliness
     and complaints;
Like Job, and Jeremiah, I struggle with
     your justice, God.
Your silence and passivity dissolution me.
I am hemmed in this long, dark tunnel
     of horrible pain.
Doubt blights my faith and apprehension
     weights my frame.

Show me your mercy and compassion so
     I am not consumed;
Quietly replace my tribulation with a
     fresh breeze of hope.
Break these chains with your gentle,
     healing power.
I will wait on the Lord and keep His way;
trusting Him with this clump of clay.

I CAN NOT TOLERATE THIS PAIN ALONE

Would you blame me, Lord,
    if you knew that sometimes
I wonder if you can hear?
Forgive me, Lord, but you
    seem to miss the essence of my prayers.

Would you find fault, Lord,
    if you knew that occasionally
I question if you have 20/20?
Forgive me, Lord, but you
    appear not to see my pain.

Would you censure me, Lord,
    if you knew that infrequently
I query if you possibly have had a stroke?
Forgive me, Lord, but you
    seem to forget to respond to my cries.

Would you doubt me, Lord,
    if you knew that once in awhile
I wonder if your taste buds are inadequate?
Forgive me, Lord, but you
    seem not to taste the salt in my tears.

FORGIVE ME LORD IF I COMPLAIN

Concrete Assurance
    God, you know all about this pain...

It's months now, Lord,

This pain and doubts of your love

Hem me in...questions...despair;
God, do you really care ?

From the sky a strong flier of rapid wing
Alighted in my yard wearing metallic green;
A wild, aquatic, handsome thing,
Before my eyes began to preen.

Thank you, Lord, a Mallard duck;
Divine providence, not just luck,
Brought reassurance of your love
Woven into life's tapestry from above.

Forgive me, Lord, if I complain;
It's just I'm so tired of this pain.
With Thanksgiving I accept this duck,
Affirmation you know about my luck.

You cared enough to send a sign;
Forgive me, Lord, when I whine.
Thank you, Lord, I feel your presence;
Your Spirit is lifting mine, in essence.

WALK THIS PATHWAY WITH ME

Lord, I hear a tumultuously violent roar;
Ominous green storm clouds gather round.
I panic trying to reach the shore;
Hold me, help me float, till on firm ground!

Lord, I feel alone; the mountain's so tall;
Menacing tenseness awaits an avalanche or mud slide.
I sense defeat by the ravines, gulches, and draws;
Tap louder, help me hear your staff as my guide!

Lord, I know the valley must come before the summit;
Dark depths of your absence weight me down so.
I ponder questions that vie to confuse my spirit.
Visit me, I call out in pain, but returns an echo!

Lord, peace ends in denial if there is no power;
   "Many are the afflictions of the
   righteous...My Spirit delivereth
   them all." (Psalms 34:19)
I feel you reach and cleanse me in this hour.
Walk with me; guide me in this pain lest I fall!

HELP ME WEATHER THIS STORM OF PAIN

Lord, my pain is like the clouds

    that are hovering all around me

        -Thunder crashing, lightening flashing-

        Ominous weather reports;

          Emergency shelters advised.

Lord, you could halt this tumultous storm

    that is assaulting and stalking my being

        -Eradicating, eliminating-

        Promise of a pain free tomorrow;

          Unshackled and unbridled.

Lord, you know this brewing, blustering storm

    that is venting rage within my body

        -Earnestly pleading and asking-

        "If not removal; stay by me,

          Help me weather the storm peacefully."

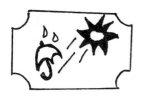

IS ANYONE ELSE HERE?

"When thou passest through the waters,
I will be with thee:
And through the rivers, they shall not
overflow thee:
When thou walkest through the fire,
Thou shalt not be burned:
Neither shall the flame kindle upon thee."

- Isaiah 43:2

JUST CALL ME ANY TIME

I called the switchboard
    and didn't get through.
I called your desk
    and a recorder answered.
I called your home
    and your phone was busy.
I called again
    and "Call Waiting" took my name.

- I waited for your return call -

The lightening flashed
    a ball of fire.
"The line is dead!"
        a repair man shouted.
The line seems spliced,
        a continuous static!
A voice cut in,
            "This number has

            has been

            disconnected11"

- I waited for your return call -

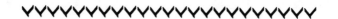

PAIN HUNGERS FOR A LIFELINE

Pain needs a lifeline
   hurled out from the ship's deck;
     A rope
       to offer a sense of hope.

Pain craves a telephone call
   dialed from a friend;
     A talk
       to arrange a short walk.

Pain longs for a card or a letter
   mailed from a well-wisher;
     A note
       to say he cared and wrote.

Pain wants a vase of flowers
   delivered from the garden;
     A fragrant smell
       to wish me well.

Pain covets a bowl of fruit
   picked from a tree;
     An apple pie
       to just say "Hi."

Pain needs a window washed
   cleaned from a ladder's height;
     An act of kindness done
       to not just come, and run.

Pain desires a floor scrubbed
   waxed from hands and knees;
      A gift of love
         to me in the Father's name above.

Pain fancies a cup of tea
   brewed in finest china;
      A muffin shared
         to show me someone cared.

Pain hungers for a lifeline
   filled with positive sanction;
      A gift of fresh options
         to dream new prospects for action.

FORGIVE ME, LORD

You know, Lord, I've laid
   prostrate before your throne;
I've asked you to search me
   and try me and reveal any wicked way.
I've studied and prayed over your words
   and petitioned your divine intervention.

And yes, Lord, I've begged, pleaded and cried!
I've beseeched you to remove this pain from me.
I've sought you in the Hymns of Faith.
I've solicited your healing and restoration.

Forgive my authoritative demand
   when I insisted you make me whole.
Forgive my impatience
   when I implored you to heal me NOW!
Forgive my doubt and disbelief
   when day turned to month and month to year.
Forgive my skepticism
   when believers enjoined me in prayer,

    - and yet the pain raged on-

Forgive my lack of conviction
   when Pastors' and Elders' prayers fell on
     deaf ears.
Forgive my wavering doubts
   when finances plummeted and still no cure.
Forgive my deepening despair
   when Christians ceased to call.
Forgive my devastated spirit
   when overwhelmed by simple tasks.

Forgive my questioning frame of mind
   when there seemed no way to escape.
Forgive my weakened disposition
   when there was no end in sight.
Forgive my continued supplication
   when you'll be busy and I'll be thinking ahead.

    -while the pain rages on-

You know, Lord, I need to ask this question;
   Will you be there to hear my entreaty?

      -or will the pain rage on-

ONLY DEATH WILL SET ME FREE

Where can I go?
Pain's my constant foe.
Where can I hide?
Respite and defeat constantly vie.

Is there no assistance?
Medicine meets resistance.
Is there no one to hear?
This torturous agony sears.

Do we not determine an animal's fate;
Cause its excruciating affliction to abate?
Why then, must I carry this cross?
Have doctors decided to treat me as dross?

Where can I flee?
Relief and solace evade me.
Where can I find hope?
The pain's so bad I can't cope!

Pray, you say?
I've tried it every day!
God chooses to ignore my plea.
Only death will set me free.

IT'S TIME
SURELY, GOD, YOU MUST OWN A WATCH

God, this pain hour by hour,
    day by day, week by week,
    year by year,
    is getting old.

Did you forget
    to set an alarm,
    or circle a date,
    in your appointment book?

Are you aware
    of beepers that can be worn
    to tell that time
    is elapsing?

Even washers and dryers,
    ovens and microwaves,
    and pill boxes,
    have buzzers.

Surely, God, you must have
    a golden time piece!
    Please have Saint Peter
    replace the Duracells!

SUPPORT GROUPS

When pain encircles me,
I know that I am not alone.
Our communication binds, yet sets me free;
Putting pain in its proper perspective zone.

We find constructive ways to deal with
anxiety and stress.
We experience a vast variety of feelings
common to chronic pain.
We have the power collectively to channel
energy, I guess.
We find shelter for our spirits, and keep
our minds sane.

We set goals to give us momentum to persist
and succeed.
We care unconditionally, accepting people
just as they are.
We give inspiration to each other to
accomplish many a deed.
We identify reasonable, small steps
taking each of us far.

We are sisters and brothers with chronic
pain.
We accept our suffering as a challenge
to endure.
We feel a peace that comes with trust,
and we all gain.
We suggest a Higher Power to alleviate fear
and composure to endure.

When pain encircles me,
I know that I am not alone.

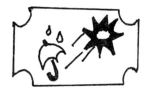

"The noontide sun is dark, and music discord, when the heart is low."

- Edward Young

"Behold, I have refined thee, but not with silver; I have chosen thee in the furnace of affliction."

- Isaiah 48:10

PAIN DEVOURS ONES SPIRIT

Pain

    Robs one

        of quality life;

    Casts one from

        a useful existence;

    Devours ones spirit

        to struggle and fight;

    Sears ones

        core, muscles, and nerves;

    Replaces confidence

        with doubt and despair;

    Erodes ones

        purpose to survive.

Pain

    Defines ones daily road;

    Dictates which avenue one must trod;
           ALONE,

    Replete of medical intervention,

        FORKLESS, Not even a choice!

      NO T'S; NO Y'S; Stuck!

      NO TURN AROUNDS; Only one way!

       NO SWITCHBACKS; Can't even turn around!

    Only hills and treacherous turns.

          SUCCUMB!

      There is no hope!

        Free at last.

COME BEFORE THE MELTING
OF THE SNOW

This pain has stripped the trees;
Icy blankets cover hard windswept ground.
Nights are clear, but freezing cold;
Icicles hang like driven swords.
Landscapes are monotonous white on white;
Wind's cold chills shiver up my spine.

Lord, please come this winter;
This pain endures the bitterness of the season.
Winter pleads for warm companionship;
Harsh blizzards blow discouragement.
God, you seem to have sealed the windows tight;
The drapes of hope and happiness are pulled.

Lord, please come this winter;
This pain causes the logs not to burn in the hearth.
Ruthless winds whip at my lonely coattails;
Cold blasts creep under every door.
Flues blow closed and smoke evades every corner;
House shakes crackle or pop in sub-zero weather.

-Darkness thickens; snow piles higher-

Lord, please come this winter;
This pain has skied its last slope.
Icy ponds bear witness to winter's frigidness;
Sleds' runners grow dull traversing the terrain.
Packed snowballs mock my pain swirling at me;
Lord, please come before the melting of the snow!

-Please come this winter-

MY SEPULCHER

A tombstone of Morning Rose,
Was the marble monument I chose;
In rustic rough-hewn sides;
For internment at the end of life's tides.

I will be buried in a plot
Shaded by a tree;
Eternal rest will be sought,
Nestled in the gentle lea.

May I have fought the good fight,
Responsive to His call;
Working and living in the Light;
Erasing every barrier or wall.

Oh Death, where is your sting?
I'm safe in my Father's arms;
Securely to my Savior I cling,
Free from this world's harms.

LORD, I'M AT THE END

Lord, I'm at the end
　of myself;
I have no strength
　nor will.
I am a pauper
　poor of spirit.

Lord, this pain is full
　of heartbreaking discouragement.
I am harrassed with pangs
　of regret and sorrow;
I have shut the door
　to my secret place.

Touch me with the freshness
　of beauty.
Fill me with rivers
　of Living Water.
Baptize me with the miracle
　of the Holy Spirit.

Lord, I surrender
　this grueling, painful feat.
I accept your gift
　of gracious peace.
I hear your voice
　of strength and pardon.

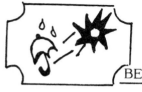

THE SUN
BEGINS TO SHINE

"These trials are
only to test your faith,
to see whether or not it is strong
and pure. It is being tested
as fire
tests gold and purifies it. Your
faith is far more precious
to God than mere gold;
so if your faith
remains strong
after being tested
and tried
in the test tube of fiery trials,
it will bring you much praise and
glory and honor
on the day of His return."

- 1 Peter 1:7

I AM EXHAUSTED BY THE TORTURE, LORD

I am troubled, Lord;
I am confused by the seeming
    turbulence you
    sovereignly
Allow to enter my life.

I am afraid, Lord;
I am worried by the intolerable
    pain you
    knowingly
Authorize hour after hour.

I am confused, Lord;
I am nauseated by the tempestuous
    waves you
    consciously
Sanction day after day.

I am worn out, Lord;
I am exhausted by the
    torture you
    constantly
Commission month after month.

I am chastised, Lord;
I am awakened by the
        steadfast hope you
        patiently
Manifest as a whisper in my ear.

I am amazed, Lord;
I am overcome by the
        peace you
        joyously
Permit to penetrate my soul.

I am quieted, Lord;
I am refreshed by the
        Living Water you
        graciously
Empower through your saving love.

I am confident, Lord;
I am less mystified by the
        pain you
        continuously
Approve year after year.

I am challenged, Lord;
I am filled by the promise of
        a new body in heaven
        assuredly
Warranted to each saint of God.

My confusion has stopped, Lord;
My doubt has turned to a
    wonder of your light
    lovingly
Confirmed by your atonement on the cross.

PROMISE OF A PAIN FREE
TOMORROW

Lord, my pain is like a tumultuous storm
    assaulting and stalking my being;
Haunting and taunting,
    brewing and deluging my soul.

Lord, you could halt this constant onslaught
    that's unshackled and unbridled;
Blustering and venting its rage,
    hacking and chipping at my faith.

Lord, control this painful storm
    quieting the ominous gales;
Hang the sun and a rainbow,
    giving promise of a pain free tomorrow.

YOU TOUCHED MY PAIN,
LORD

I sang hymns of faith
   through my tears.
I sang hymns of faith
   through my pain.
I sang hymns of faith
   through my loneliness.

I had forgotten the words,
   you brought them to my lips.
I had forgotten the words,
   you spoke them to my soul.
I had forgotten the words,
you selected them to meet my needs.

I felt you come
   and bring peace to my heart.
I felt you come
   and pour out reassurance.
I felt you come
   and touch my pain, Lord.

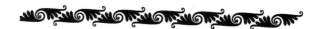

THE PAIN WILL BE OVER

Today, Lord, you knew
My heart was weighted and heavy
My spirit arid and dry
My faith tried and tested

Today, Lord, I know
Your heart felt my burden
Your spirit instilled new resolve
Your promise demonstrated boldness
for high in its tree
in the nearby swamp
confidentially perched,
our majestic Bald Eagle,
a sign of your
celestial assurance

Today, Lord, I know
This enveloping pain will be over
All exhausting tests interpreted
Prescriptions issued by the Great Physician

Today, Lord, I know
The Eagle returned
The Eagle soared freely
The Eagle reflected your grace
The pain will be over

"When thou art in tribulation,
and all these things are come
upon you...If thou shalt turn
to the Lord God, and shalt be obedient
unto His voice; He will not forsake thee."

— Deuteronomy 4:30-31

"And God shall wipe away all tears from
their eyes; and there shall be no more
death, neither sorrow, nor crying, neither
shall there be any more pain."

— Revelations 21:4

"These things have I spoken to you, that
in Me you may have peace. In the world
you have tribulation, but take courage:
I have overcome the world."

— John 16:33

"Wherefore I desire that ye
faint not at my
tribulation for you."

— Ephesians 3:14

MAKE ME A PEARL

Keep me alert, probing, questioning, keen;
Bind me in spirit
    so your presence can easily be seen.
Help me learn to trust your plans for my life more;
As a victor in Christ, keep me committed to the core.

Challenge me to become more intimate with Him;
Fill me with courage, serenity,
    and acceptance up to the rim.
Give me a new song and be in charge all my day;
Keep my fruit sweet for all to eat that come my way.

Make me a pearl if I must endure this awful pain;
Pierce me with the grains of sand
    so healing will be my gain.
Test my endurance, for I will finish the race;
Cash in my passport as I reach that heavenly place.

FRAGRANCE OF A VIOLET

God has a plan in mind
    for any disappointment I face;
    - The bondage of bitterness -
    is set free with "FORGIVENESS,
    ...the fragrance the violet sheds
    on the heel that crushed it."
                    (Mark Twain)

During bewildering times
    when I don't understand
    - God is still who He says He is -
    and will do what He
    promises in His word;
    I am acceptant, not resigned.

Even in this painful and
    inescapable circumstance,
    - it is well with my soul -
    God is at work in my life
    to do something for my good
    and His glory.

I choose to live authentically
    and practice hopefulness
    -putting my faith in God -
    who has the power
    to take this trial and
    turn it into a blessing.

God loves me with an
    unwavering, unconditional love
    - that is weatherproofed -
    to dispel all of life's storms.
    His hand is soverign in my life,
    even when life hurts.

ACCEPTANCE

Waking in the night,
a
reverberating
resounding
Ringing cadence;
surging
rushing
heightening
of the breakers of Lake Superior
-just outside the cabin door-
bringing
peace
calm
sereneness
acquiescence.
I wish to stay,
but
Now, I can let go.

Your sonorous oscillation and pulsation
Wield lathery, frothy spume
Against the jagged, resolute boulders
Lining your grandiose shorelines;
While all the time,
Your undulations glisten like diamonds
Glittering, and penetrating the window
of my retreat;
Heightening the
still
placid
Silent calm
Settling in my soul.
Now,
I can let go.

PAIN IS AN OPEN WINDOW

Pain is an open window
  to discern things of the heart;
    -A Saviour-
Who promises to go with me through
  the valley;
    -A Minister-
Who provides warm pastoral care;
    -A Quiet Time-
Which confers food to my soul;
    -An Undershepherd-
Who extends God in the skin.

Pain is an open window
  to see what is important;
    -A Faithful Husband-
Who loves me unconditionally;
    -A Steadfast Friend-
Who stands by my side;
    -A Loyal Lover-
Who respects my mutual needs;
    -A Devoted Laborer-
Who works to provide unwaveringly.

Pain is an open window
    to enjoy our Creator's handiwork;
      -A Bright Red Cardinal-
Which alights in the nearest tree;
      -A Hummingbird-
Which hovers at the nectar feeder;
      -A Red Squirrel-
Which raps and begs at the patio door;
      -A Bald Eagle-
Which perches atop an old dead tree.

Pain is an open window
    to recognize skills and talents;
      -A Water, or Oil Painting-
Which captures life's experiences;
      -A Sewing or Craft Project-
Which finishes a creative challenge;
      -A Decorated Cake or Recipe Tried-
Which behold the joy shared with family;
      -A Letter Written, or a Gift Sent-
Which "visit" with a special touch.

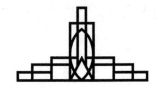

CONFIRM YOUR PEACE THROUGH HEALING

Lord of the heavens, my Lord,
  come in your power and might.
Surround me with your angels,
  take authority tonight.
Prepare me and create optimum healing,
  hear and intervene,
    while I am kneeling.

I raise my soul in prayer
  to implore your presence.
I raise my hands in reverence
  to praise you for you are holy.
I raise my voice in song
  to uplift your name in melody.

I raise my petitions in supplication
  to confirm your power and authority.
I raise my face in openness
  to erase any hidden or secret thing.
I raise my faith in childlike fervor
  to receive your peace
    and power through healing.

IN THE FURNACE

The thirsty flames are invisible, Lord.
Intense heat is inescapably chaining
   me to this chord.
I stand melting in this blistering
   furnace pit;
Feeling desolate, with silent warfare
   defying my wit.

My soul groans and cries out,
"It makes no sense; illogical, I hear
   myself shout!
I'm trapped like a rat in a darkened
   sewer pipe;
I refuse to surrender to the pain! I'm
   not the type!"

Pain, struggles, and confusion seem unfair
But Jesus never sinned, yet He had
   suffering to bear.
Insults, hardships, persecutions made
   Paul weak;
He asked three times for healing, and
   contentment did he seek.

Declaring God's absolute sovereignty,
   like Job, he rested his case.
Wow! Job's avalanche is not something
   that I want to face!
How shortsighted! I must die obediently
   to self;
Accept my circumstances; put fear and
   and apprehension on the shelf.

Lord, refine, purify, reshape, and
   temper me.
Soften and penetrate my heart as pleasing
   unto Thee.
Strengthen me to endure what you've called
   me to do;
Help me build patience, and persevere
   through heartache too.

I place my pain on the altar and raise
   my hands in surrender.
Incline my heart to understanding, new
   vision and strength render.
Make me real, quiet, supportive, and
   available to be used of Thee;
Fill me with compassion, and let me an
   encouragement be.

As the flames lick up around me, I'll
   leave the future to Him.
He is omniscient and sees forever, while
   my eyesight is rather dim.
I'll accept and trust completely, rather
   than trying to explain;
I'll accept the tribulation with good
   cheer, trying not to complain.

CONTEMPLATION

Lost in thought
   Contemplation
   Contentment
Waves communicating
   with my soul;
Lapping, clapping
      Peace
      Quiet
      Calm
All is well with my soul;
Oh, my God, how great
      Thou Art!

STILL WILL I TRUST

Deceitful, unjust men
  insult and mock my pain
    - as if to say -
    "Just where is your God?"
    "Where is your help?"

Waves and billows of pain
  and this burning trial
    - wash over me -
    I acknowledge allowance
    by your hand.

Judge me, oh God,
  and plead my case
    - send the light -
    Illuminate the truth;
    Deliver me from oppression.

If earth holds no balm
  for my healing
    - still will I trust -
    God has redeemed me;
    I am His child.

God is the light of my hope
  He will make a way
    - through the darkest times -
    My faith is deeper than
    this burning circumstance.

I will again find hope
  and praise my Savior
    - In the shadow of His wings -
    will I abide until
    life's trials are o'er.
                (Psalms 42,43,63)

DON'T LET TOMORROW ROB TODAY

Quiet my worries about tomorrow;
Grant me strength to get through today.
Release me from things that torment and
    harrow;
Erase from me fears that burden and weigh.

Dry my tear stained face;
I need you in the flesh today.
Send me equipped by your grace;
Nourish me and lead the way.

Bring to my lips songs of faith;
Ingrain on my mind verses from your Book.
Clarify to my ears just what it sayeth;
Quench my thirst at The Living Brook.

Receive my life to do your will;
Form images of hope for the future.
Instill courage to contribute still;
Reveal your lamb that needs my nurture.

DIAMONDS IN THE ROUGH

Standing here in the furnace
  we are reminded that
      diamonds
  are chunks of coal
under lengthy duress,
as the watchman feeds the fire
  shovel after shovel full.

We are powerless to stop
  the ensuing heat,
    but
  are tempered
to find strength to cope
    and
achieve inner tranquility.

With our faith sharpened,
We try to recognize the
  intended goals
by the light of the flames;
    Confident
  We will find refuge
In Your reassuring embrace.

The ability to retain hardness
at a red heat
enhances
the value of diamonds
as tools;
freeing us to be used in
God's ultimate purpose for our lives.

A diamond has an indestructible
quality;
We too will find a way
to transcend our pain;
All cooled, refreshed, and polished;
God is in charge.

- A vital reality -

ACCEPT MY PRAYERS TODAY,
LORD

Please...

Give me strength to cope
Open my heart to your promises
Help me overcome my fears
Place positive thoughts in my mind
Move me to have positive actions
Administer healing to my body and spirit
Safeguard me and cast out the whisperings
    of darkness
Visit me and cleanse me from all unrigh-
    teousness
Transmit your love even through this pain
Draw me personally closer to my creator
Equip me to endure this pain's wrath
Supply me with patience, stamina, and
    courage
Reduce stress-producing interactions,
    circumstances, and perceptions
Let me drink in hope even when my pain
    can not be fixed
Change my attitude from the submission to
    pain, to wise management of the pain
Comfort me when new treatments prove
    inadequate
Hold my umbrella when doubts rain down
    upon my spirit
Lighten this heavy cross with loving
    good friends
Assist me to mourn each loss, and the
    limited energy span
Teach me to adapt, and accept, what I
    can, and can not do
Enrich me with today's happiness despite
    the pain

Make me deaf to myths, misconceptions, and
    false rainbows of treatment
Provide me the vision to prioritize, pace,
    and participate as fully as possible
Show me that you'll stay near by and
    love me through this pain
Deepen my faith to believe your word,
    and to trust you more fully
Let me absorb your love, light, and truth
    in the darkness of this hour
Accept my obedience and quieted question-
    ing in solitude with you
Commission me to tend your flock, even
    through this pain

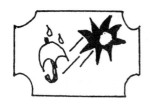

P. S.

_____

"To get back on your feet,
miss two car payments."
(Unknown)

"No one can make you feel
inferior without your consent."
(Eleanor Roosevelt)

"Patience is power;
with time and patience the
mulberry leaf becomes silk."
(Chinese Proverb)

A COLLECTION OF REASONS THAT WELL-MEANING PEOPLE GIVE FOR THE CAUSALITY OF CHRONIC PAIN, OR CHRONIC ILLNESS

Some people would say that pain or illness is:

- An alarm, or buzzer going off, signaling that a part of our physical being is in distress and needs repair.

- A genetic factor, or a hereditary predisposition to a given disease or condition.

- The suppression of the immune system when the intimate connection between emotional, mental, spiritual, and physical health is out of kilter.

- An injury, accident, or environmental issue.

- God-appointed instruction ready to stretch and challenge us.

- A growth experience in a deeper walk with Christ.

- A time of groundedness to learn to know that God is real.

- A time of discipline, but not a period of God's displeasure.

- To demonstrate our weakness for then, as it was true for the apostle Paul, we are made strong.

- A messenger from Satan to hurt, bother, and buffet us.

- To create confusion, but that growth and wisdom await us.

- A demanding and humiliating experience to make us obedient and dependent on Christ.

- To teach us to be well-contented in whatever circumstance.

- An inherited "original sin" to cause us suffering, illness, and death.

- A relationship between personal sins and sickness, while others are quick to point out that many who live upright lives are also often times ill.

-Suffering in our bodies so that we become patient in consolation so others may be comforted when in trouble and affliction.

-Necessary so we would never again trust in our self, but only in God, as a partaker of Christ's suffering and His glory.

-To fulfill God's purpose to bring us to the point of giving up - yet to come forth with the gentleness of Christ rejoicing, having proven God faithful.

-God's intention so that when He delivers us from this pain, we will never again doubt His power to deliver us in every present and future trial.

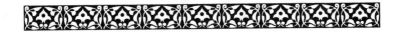

SUBJECT TITLE INDEX

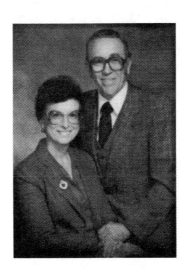

I am pressed beyond endurance and unable to understand, and to control this pain. No longer will I struggle to figure it out. I have come to the end of my own strength. My eyes are on the Lord to give grace and strength to persevere with an obedient heart to do His will; knowing that to do so is the surest path to peace. The battle is no longer mine. I trust God to end this suffering rather it be by life, or death; in His own time, and in His own way.

Priscilla Olson and her husband Gordon reside in rural Wyoming, Minnesota.

For additional copies, contact your local book stores, or if desired order directly by mail below:

Ship to: (Please Print)

Name _____

Address_____

City, State, and 9-digit zip

_____

_____

Day Phone _____

____ Copies of IN THE FURNACE
     $8.95 each

____ $2.50 Postage per book
     if ordering by mail

____ .45 Minnesota Sales Tax

_____

____ Total Amount En-
     closed

Fundraising opportunity avail-able for church, and non-profit organizations.

Make checks payable to:
     IN THE FURNACE

Send to: Priscilla Olson
         28425 Forest Blvd. N.
         Wyoming, MN 55092-9339
         (612) 462-3436